TABLE OF CONTENTS

AROMATHERAPHY 23

THE MOST POPULAR ESSENTIAL OILS FOR BEGINNERS 45

STORING ESSENTIAL OILS...................... 82

INTRODUCTION

Essential oils are extracts from natural plant materials. They retain the plant's scent as well as the plant's therapeutic properties. This is commonly also called the plant's "essence". These oils are a highly concentrated extract of the plant they came from.

The production of essential oils is most commonly done by steam distillation of the plant materials. Another common method is cold pressing of materials, or solvent extraction to gain the valuable oils.

Essential oils found in many different plants, especially the aromatic plants, vary in odor and flavor, which are governed by the types and amount of constituents present in oils. Additionally, the amount of essential oil from different plants is different and this determines the price of essential oil. Apart from aromatic compounds, indigenous pigments contribute to varying colors of essential oil. This can affect the applications as the ingredient in some particular foods. Essential oils have been known to possess antioxidant and antimicrobial activities, thereby serving as natural additives in foods and food products. It can be used as active compounds in packaging materials, in which the properties of those materials, particularly water vapor barrier property associated with hydrophobicity in nature of essential oils, can be improved. Almost any part of a plant may be the source of the oil, which could be extracted and fully exploited for food applications or others. Modern technologies have been continuously developed to conquer the limitation of conventional methods, and to enhance the extraction efficacy. Due to the increasing attention in natural additives, essential oils from several plants have been used more widely, especially in conjunction with other preservations under concept of "hurdle technology." Thus, essential oils can serve as the alternative additives or processing aid as green technology. Essential oils are used in the alternative medicine of aromatherapy.

ESSENTIAL OILS

What Is An Essential Oil?

Essential oils, also called volatile odoriferous oil, are aromatic oily liquids extracted from different parts of plants, for example, leaves, peels, barks, flowers, buds, seeds, and so on. They can be extracted from plant materials by several methods, steam distillation, expression, and so on. Among all methods, for example, steam distillation method has been widely used, especially for commercial scale production.

What Is A "100% Pure" Oil

The term "pure" has been used almost as a replacement for "single" essential oil. This means that pure essential oils are single oils (such as Lavender, Tea Tree,

Rosemary, etc.) – and not a blend or synergy mix of aromatherapy oils.

A 100% pure essential oil means that you're purchasing just that oil, and not an essential oil blend or a bottle that has oil blended together with carrier oils or other additives. I would go as far to say that "100% pure" wouldn't be advertised for oils that could possibly contain additives, fillers, or chemical aromas.

However, companies might walk the fine line and call their single oils "pure oils" (without the 100% part), and possibly have some fillers or other chemical substances mixed into their oils. Who knows! Again, there is no 3rd party that polices this term, so it should on its own also not be your sole criteria for trusting any essential oil brand of choice. The only real way to know whether or not any essential oil bottle (or company) is trustworthy, consistent and accurate in their sales and advertising, is to go as far as looking at chemical test results of oil batches and bottles, and pick a brand that readily discloses this information for the public to see.

Are Essential Oils The Same As Fragrances Or Aromatic Oils?

Essential oils are not the same as perfume or fragrance oils, which are also called aromatic oils or aroma oils. Perfume oils are artificially created in a chemist's lab, while essential oils are a product of nature.

Fragrances are made to mimic an otherwise natural smell (such as "spring rain" fragrances). Of course, the synthetically created fragrance products do not offer the therapeutic benefits that the actual essential oils offer.

Only pure essential oils should be used for aromatherapy purposes.

However, fragrance oils do have their place and applications. They are widely available and quite inexpensive to obtain, and are commonly used in soap making, candle making, or perfumes and cosmetics.

Where Do Essential Oils Come From?

The earth is filled with different plants that play a vital role in producing oxygen, food, creating habitats and regulating water.

Within the seeds, stems, bark, roots, wood, needles, flowers and fruit of these wonderful plants, essential oils can be found.

For thousand of years people have been using plant parts for health solutions, beauty treatments, religious ceremonies and burials.

So, if you have ever wondered where essential oils come from... they are all around us.

The amount of essential oil each plant produces varies greatly depending on many factors. Some include the time of day, the time of year, climate and environmental conditions.

How Does Essential Oils Help Plants?

Essential oils are found in different parts of living plants. Essential oils will vary from plant to plant, or species to species. Here are some ways they may help plants:

• Give a plant its distinct smell

- Protect plants by keeping insects and pests away.

- Play a role in plant pollination

- Resist microbial attack

- Assist during periods of low nutrition

- Protect against temperature extremes

- Helps the plant heal itself when injured

How Are Essential Oils Made?

There are several methods for extracting essential oils from plants. Each method requires care and caution to extract only the highest quality essential oil. This ensures that the natural benefits of the plants are preserved.

Producing a high quality essential oil starts with the right timing.

For example, jasmine must be harvested at early in the morning in order to preserve its aromatic compounds, before the buds have fully opened. Once they have blossomed, the flowers rapidly loss their aromatic compounds.

It is crucial that the correct plant part is harvested when preparing a plant for distillation.

The Corandrum sativum plant produces 2 kinds of essential oils that are completely different in chemical makeup. One is cilantro essential oil, it is derived from the leaves of the plant. Coriander is the other, it is derived from the seeds of the plant.

Once the plant part has been harvested, the distillation process must start quickly before the plant loses its potency. The distillation process separates the essential oils from the plant part to make a usable oil.

The most common essential oil extraction methods are steam distillation and cold pressed (aka expression).

With steam distillation, heated steam and pressure are used to separate essential oils from their plant parts.

Cold pressing is another popular distillation method. Typically it is used to produce citrus essential oils from the rinds and peels of citrus fruits.

Did you know it takes approximately 50 grapefruit peels to create one 15 ml bottle of the essential oil?

Some other essential oil extraction methods are CO2 extracted oils and solvent extracted absolutes.

Cutting corners during any part of the production process may result in a lower quality essential oil. A lower quality oil will be less effective and may even be harmful.

Why Is It Important For Essential Oils To Be Tested?

Once essential oils have been carefully created, they must go through a quality check for these main goals:

• Verify potency

• Ensure purity

Two common test essential oils should go through are gas chromatography and mass spectrometry to help producers analyze essential oil composition and chemical makeup.

If you have an oil brand that you buy from, the company should have these tests available on their website or per customer request.

Gas chromatography (GC) identifies what chemical compounds are in each essential oil and the level they appear.

Mass spectometry (MS) analyzes the makeup to identify the different aromatic compounds of an essential oil.

Once an essential oil batch has been thoroughly tested to ensure that it is pure and potent without fillers or containments that would effect the quality or safety of the oil.

Unfortunately, not all essential oil companies follow the meticulous process that is required to offer high quality essential oils. Cutting costs, saving time and not testing produce poor quality oil.

What Is A Carrier Oil?

Carrier oils carry the essential oils into the skin, this means you can use less essential oil. This saves you money but does not lessen the effectiveness of the essential oil. Isn't that wonderful!

Plus, adding a carrier oil also gives you all the benefits that the carrier oil offers. So now you can see why diluting essential oils is a no brainer right?

Lets recap the 6 benefits of diluting essential oils with a carrier oil:

• Essential oils evaporate way slower, giving them time to absorb

• Lessens chance of skin reactions or irritations

• Saves you money because less essential oil drops are needed

• Makes spreading them on skin easier

• Improves the effectiveness of essential oils

• You get the added benefits the carrier oil offers

Here are some carrier oils that can be used:

• Jojoba oil (wax)

• Sweet Almond Oil

• Grapeseed Oil

• Virgin Coconut Oil

• Fractionated Coconut Oil

• Argan Oil

- Rosehip Oil

- Avocado Oil

- Shea Butter

Where Do I Apply Essential Oils?

Essential oils can be applied to almost every body part with a few exceptions. You must avoid eyes, inner ears, inside nose, or other orifices.

Also remember that facial tissue is delicate so use caution when applying oils to face and be sure to dilute well before using.

Apply essential oils to the location where you need them. Have a sore neck? Massage them onto neck. Upset tummy? Apply to abdomen. Yes... it really is that simple. Always remember to dilute too.

If using for the aromatic benefits, you can apply to chest or wrists. Like if using lavender before bedtime to help you sleep, mix 1-2 drops in a teaspoon of jojoba oil and apply to upper chest. You will be able to inhale the aroma and fall asleep fast.

How should I use essential oils?

• Aromatically

Essential oils are best known for their aromas, which can help create an environment to suit your specific needs. In addition to adding them to cleaning products and beauty staples, you can infuse the air directly with your favorite fragrance by using one of our many diffusers. These handy aroma atomizers can be placed anywhere you crave a fresh scent.

• Topically

Many essential oils have skin-enhancing benefits and can be applied directly to the skin or added to your existing beauty products. You can also combine them with a carrier oil or your daily moisturizer for easy application.

• Internally

AROMATHERAPHY

What is Aromatherapy?

Aromatherapy may promote relaxation and help relieve stress. It has also been used to promote sleep, support overall health and wellness and it may even help support healthy blood pressure.

Aromatherapy uses oils extracted from flowers, seeds, leaves, roots, fruit and twigs for special effect. These essential oils are formulated to work in harmony with the body and may have an ability to affect a person's well-being.

Derived from the parts of plants or trees, essential oils possess a complex nature that is difficult to reproduce outside of nature. In fact, some oils contain substances that don't occur anywhere else naturally.

Aromatherapy History

Essential oils have been used for thousands of years as stimulants, sedatives, and for religious and medicinal purposes. Aromatherapy is the century-old practice of using volatile plant oils, also referred to as essential oils, to support overall health and well-being.

It is part of the holistic healing spectrum that, in addition to essential oils, also utilizes other natural ingredients like vegetable oils, jojoba (a liquid wax), herbs, sea salts, clays and muds.

Aromatherapists apply some aromatherapy oils directly to the skin via aromatherapy massages, but they also use the oils to freshen the air of their living spaces via sprays or essential oil diffusers.

The oils can also be inhaled directly, although one should be careful not to swallow or consume the liquid oils.

"Practitioners of aromatherapy believe that fragrances in the oils stimulate nerves in the nose. Those nerves send impulses to the part of the brain that controls memory and emotion. Depending on the type of oil [the scent], the result on the body may be calming or stimulating."

Health Benefits of Aromatherapy

Take a whiff of the air around you. What do you smell? Are you immediately put in a good mood with the smell of fresh cut flowers? Suddenly craving pie with the smell of baked apples and cinnamon wafting through the halls? Or feel like gagging after being blasted with exhaust from the bus?

It's easy to see how our sense of smell impacts our feelings. The sense of smell is incredibly powerful. Your body can distinguish more than 1 trillion different scents. But, aromatherapy isn't just about appealing smells; it also offers many potential health benefits including the following:

• Supporting relaxation and stress relief

• Aiding mood and well being

• Supporting immune system and circulatory health.

Aromatherapy can be a great, natural, complementary health treatment in a variety of situations.

How to Buy Essential Oils

To purchase quality essential oils that are best suited for your particular needs and budget, there are a number of important factors to keep in mind. Read the below important tips to learn what you need to know when comparing essential oils offered from different retailers, wholesalers and other sources:

• At first, some individuals are understandably leery of purchasing essential oils online. Be assured that there are many reputable essential oil and aromatherapy retailers and suppliers that sell their essential oils online. Buying online gives you the opportunity to shop with many more reputable companies than if you were limited to only those businesses within your locale. Reputable companies are experts in properly bottling and packaging their oils for shipment.

• When shopping for essential oils, watch out for words such as "fragrance oil," "nature identical oil," or "perfume oil." These words indicate that what you see is not a pure, single essential oil. I've seen companies label fragrance oils (that can be combinations of essential oils and chemicals or just plain chemicals) and perfume oils as being suitable for aromatherapy. This is a tipoff that the vendor knows little about aromatherapy. Beginners need to watch out for retailers/suppliers who inaccurately use the term aromatherapy for their own sales gain.

• Be precautious of suppliers that promote their essential oils as being "therapeutic grade" or "aromatherapy grade." There is no governmental regulating body that grades or certifies essential oils as "therapeutic grade" or "aromatherapy grade." Not all companies use these terms with any form of deception in mind, but some may. Therefore, it's important to understand the background behind this terminology and evaluate these suppliers based on other factors and the tips shown below.

• The term "pure essential oil" is also a term overused in the aromatherapy industry. The term can clue you in that at least the retailer/supplier is aware of the importance of seeking out pure oils, but don't rely solely on a vendor's use of the term "pure" when deciding to purchase. Pure essential oils can be distilled from poor quality crops, be sitting in someone's inventory or on a store's shelves for years, be stored in a way that damages the oils, or be mishandled by vendors so that oils are accidentally mixed during bottling. So, don't get overly impressed by a vendor that labels their oils as "pure."

• Most vendors selling quality oils at sizes of 4 oz. Or smaller sell their oils in dark colored glass. Be leery of vendors that sell oils at these sizes in plastic or clear glass containers.

• When purchasing oils online, it is not uncommon for larger sizes of essential oils to be shipped in non-glass containers to avoid breakage and reduce shipping fees. Essential oils, however, can dissolve plastic bottles and the quality of the oil can deteriorate more rapidly. When receiving oils shipped in plastic or clear glass, be sure to immediately transfer the essential oils to dark colored glass bottles, unless you plan to use the essential oil (i.e. formulate with it) immediately. It's a savvy idea to keep empty bottles on hand. If you purchase from a supplier that ships in plastic, ask them how long the oil has been stored in the plastic bottles prior to shipment. Ideally, you want to work with suppliers that transfer to plastic just prior to shipment.

- Some vendors also sell larger quantities of oil in aluminum bottles. Aluminum is said to be acceptable if the inside of the bottle is lined.

- Avoid purchasing or storing essential oils that are packaged in bottles that include rubber eyedropper bulbs in the top. Over time, essential oils are strong enough to dissolve the rubber dropper and contaminate the oil. Instead, small retail sizes of essential oils tend to be sold in bottles that include an orifice reducer , sometimes known as a euro dropper, that is made out of a material that won't contaminate the oils. If essential oils are packaged or stored in bottles that do not include an orifice reducer, a pipette can be used to dispense essential oils by the drop. Larger sizes of essential oils tend to be packaged without orifice reducers because larger bulk sizes of essential oils tend to be purchased by those that prepare larger recipes and measuring by the drop would be inappropriate for them.

• Seek out vendors that provide detailed information about their oils and that give you confidence in their knowledge and background. Pay attention to the educational background that they provide and their length of time in business.

• If you are comparing online vendors, send e-mail to them asking questions that you have. If you don't have any, think of something to ask so that you have a reason to write them.

• Watch out for vendors that sell each of their "essential oils" for the same price. This doesn't guarantee that the oils are not pure or of good quality, but it really does scream of concern. Generally speaking, Neroli, Jasmine and Rose, for instance, should cost a lot more than Geranium and Ylang Ylang and anyone reputable in selling essential oils should realize that and should be aware that selling all oils for the same price is a red flag to knowledgeable consumers. A good quality Patchouli usually costs more than Eucalyptus. The basic, common citrus oils including Sweet Orange oils are some of the least expensive oils.

• When buying essential oils locally, watch for oils that have dust on the top of the bottles or boxes. This is an indication that the oils have been sitting around. As time passes, most oils oxidize, lose their therapeutic properties, and their aroma diminishes. The bottles should be sealed so that the oil couldn't be contaminated by other customers. The one advantage to purchasing oils in person is that they often provide "tester" bottles so that you can evaluate the aroma. Keep in mind, however, that the essential oil in the testers don't necessarily reflect the exact aroma of the oil you will receive as the tester bottles are more prone to oxidation due to the number of times the bottles are opened and closed. Also, the testers aren't always from the same lot.

• While I frequently shop and support a number of health food stores in my area and don't want to discourage anyone from supporting their local holistic health related stores, the products that are glaringly absent from my shopping cart at health food stores are essential or carrier oils. I'm not a fan of purchasing essential oils in health food stores as the oils don't sell very quickly and have more risk of aging/oxidizing while sitting on their shelves. Additionally, the brands generally sold in health food stores (but not always) tend to be lower quality oils or risk being stored in less than optimal ways (i.e. when they aren't on the shelf, are they stored in a hot storage area that can be detrimental to the oil). There certainly are exceptions, but health store owners and their staff generally just don't know as much about essential oils as retailers and suppliers that specialize in essential oils and aromatherapy, often with owners that have actively and formally studied and worked with the oils.

• Avoid buying oils from retailers/suppliers that don't provide the essential oil's botanical name (Latin name), country of origin or method of extraction. I've bought good quality oils from companies that don't bother listing this information (though I contact them to confirm this information prior to purchase), but I often wonder why any truly knowledgeable vendor would not realize the importance of automatically including this information.

For instance, there are multiple varieties of Bay, Cedarwood, Chamomile, Eucalyptus, and so on. Each offers different therapeutic properties. The country of origin for oils is also important because the climate and soil conditions can affect the resulting properties of the oil. Is that rose oil steam distilled or is it an absolute? Any good aromatherapy vendor should realize the necessity for providing this information.

• Several corporations sell essential oils via MLM and distributor arrangements. It is understandable that you may want to trust every statement and suggestion that your beloved best friend, relative or even that "honest" friend from church may tell you about the essential oils that he/she is so excitedly trying to sell you as a distributor. Essential oils offer many impressive benefits. If the claims you hear sound too good to be true, however, it's ok for you to be skeptical. Be prudent. Be careful. It is safest to do your own independent homework using multiple sources, and confirm usage and safety information first.

• Be very careful purchasing essential oils from Amazon. I shop on Amazon for particular things, but not for essential oils or carrier oils. At the time that I am writing this, I do not believe that Amazon does anything to "verify" the authenticity or quality of the essential oil brands that they sell. Even for oils that have amazing ratings. Having said that, I want to be clear that I don't mean to imply that every brand or essential oil that is sold via Amazon is adulterated. I do know of at least one highly respected brand of essential oils that does offer their oils through Amazon (in addition to selling them through their own website). My point is to express that there is reason to be very diligent and very careful if considering buying essential oils through Amazon.

• Educate yourself about the FDA guidelines for essential oils and aromatherapy products.

• Organic oils are typically superior to non-organic oils.

• Be careful when buying essential oils from companies that primarily sell to the food & beverage or perfumery industries. Some vendors that primarily sell to these industries may have different goals in the purchase and sale of their essential oils than the goals of vendors that sell oils specifically for therapeutic aromatherapy use. The restaurant and perfumery industries typically desire essential oils that have a standardized (consistent) aroma or flavor. The oils sold by these sources may be redistilled to remove or add specific constituents (natural chemicals found in the oils). These re-distillations or adulterations are generally not as beneficial. However, it can be tempting to shop with such vendors as their prices can be cheaper. If desiring to buy from such a vendor, inquire first to ask about their methods.

• Most of us need to watch how much we spend. It's very tempting to buy essential oils from the companies that sell them for the lowest price. Price alone isn't an indication of quality, but it can be. Knowledgeable vendors that spend countless hours locating quality oils, pay the expensive fees to test their oils (refer to the links available towards the bottom of the page to learn more about essential oil testing) and provide the results to customers and provide free samples upon request should rightfully be charging more for their essential oils than retailers that stock oils that they've sourced from the cheapest sources.

• When choosing to try a particular vendor, place a small first order and ask for asamples (don't ask for a sample of everything, honestly ask for 2-4 samples of oils that you are sincerely interested in purchasing). The goal is to find out if this is a vendor that you are pleased with without wasting your money on large orders that you might not be happy with.

• It is costly and time consuming for vendors to provide samples. Some vendors and suppliers receive an overwhelming number of requests for free samples. It can be hard for vendors to determine legitimate and honest sample requests from those just looking for freebies and that have no intention of ever placing a future order. Therefore, some vendors do need to charge a small fee for providing samples. These policies should not reflect poorly on the vendor.

• Be cautious about purchasing oils from traveling vendors that set up shop at street fairs, farmer's markets, craft shows, festivals or other limited-time events. Some traveling vendors at these events may know their customers have no recourse against them after the event is over. I want to be very careful here as there indeed are highly reputable, experienced sellers at such events, and some vendors do have a well respected, strong, local and permanent presence in the area of the show/festival. This is a caution for beginners who are not able to reliably judge quality at first, and I trust that experienced, honest vendors understand this precaution. When considering a purchase, ask the vendor for details about their experience and where their business is physically located.

Ethical and experienced vendors are generally happy to answer detailed questions about their products/oils and tend to fully respect the importance of qualifying questions. They should be be more than happy to share their background with you.

How to Choose the Best Essential Oils

The most important factor in choosing essential oils is to make sure that they are 100% pure. There is no standardized grading system for essential oils, and no authority board in the United States (or really, anywhere in the world) that oversees the oils. Some companies may refer to their products as "therapeutic grade" or "Grade A", but they are simply assigning these to their own products and it is not overseen by any governing body.

Your best bet is to do some of your own research on a brand or company to find out how they source their oils. Reputable companies should provide their consumers with test results (such as Gas Chromatograph/Mass Spectrometer or GC/MS) that verify purity. This ensures that the oils have not been mixed with synthetic additives or diluted in any way. If you can't get this information from a company, you probably don't want their products. But even then, you have to trust that the results you are given are legitimate.

The question of organic essential oils can be a bit confusing because, again, there is no board of authority that oversees the growth of plants that are used for essential oils. Most reputable companies choose plant suppliers who farm without pesticides, even if they are not specifically 'certified' because of differences in international rules.

When choosing the best essential oils, it all comes down to finding a trusted brand. And don't be fooled—the most expensive brand of oils is not always the best! Sometimes they are just higher priced. This is especially true if they come from companies who use a pyramid selling plan with local representatives. Buying your essential oils online (after doing some research about the company) is probably the best and most affordable way to source them.

THE MOST POPULAR ESSENTIAL OILS FOR BEGINNERS

Here are some of the most popular essential oils that you can find on the market today. And there's a reason everyone loves them—because they're amazing! These must-have essential oils for beginners are in the cabinets of every EO guru you'll ever meet. And you may find that they carry these oils around with them wherever they go.

1. Lavender Essential Oil

2. Peppermint Essential Oil

3. Lemon Essential Oil

4. Eucalyptus Essential Oil

5. Frankincense Essential Oil

6. Tea Tree Essential Oil

7. Chamomile Essential Oil

8. Rosemary Essential Oil

9. Patchouli Essential Oil

10. Sweet Orange Essential Oil

11. Marjoram Essential Oil

12. Grapefruit Essential Oil

13. Cinnamon Essential Oil

14. Clove Essential Oil

15. Clary Sage Essential Oil

1. Lavender Essential Oil

Lavandula angustofolia

This must-have essential oil for beginners is effective for so many different uses. The floral scent makes it one of the best smelling essential oils that is beloved by many. Although this oil is known for being mild and calming, a few people are allergic so it's important to take care.

Useful for:

• Relaxation

• Skin issues

• Speeding healing

• Improved digestion

• Pain relief

• Reduced inflammation

Application:

While most essential oils need to be diluted with a carrier oil, Lavender is safe to apply directly to the skin. For promoting healthy sleep, add a few drops to a diffuser and place in the bedroom before sleep. You can also diffuse it into a room for a calming scent that reaches the whole family.

2. Peppermint Essential Oil

Mentha piperita

One of the best smelling essential oils that almost everyone loves, Peppermint offers a myriad of health benefits as well as a boost of energy. Its minty scent is reminiscent of candy canes and fresh summer days.

Useful for:

• Alleviating headaches

• Relieving digestive issues such as gas or heartburn

• Reduces feelings of stress and anxiety

• Kills germs (particularly in the mouth)

• Freshens air

• Cooling and refreshing

• Removes redness and irritating skin issues

• Helps with congestion

Application:

Use in a cool mist humidifier during winter months for fighting colds and cleaning the air. Add a drop to a glass of water and use as a mouthwash. Place a few drops with a carrier oil and massage into sore or tired muscles.

3. Lemon Essential Oil

Citrus Limonum

Who doesn't associate the smell of lemons with something fresh and clean?! It takes about 50 lemons to make a small 15ml bottle of essential oil—and you can tell just by opening it.

Useful for:

• Freshening air

• Killing germs in kitchens and bathrooms

• Aiding with digestion

• Reducing pain (arthritis, gout)

• Healing skin

• Promoting immune system

• Increasing energy and uplifting the mood

• Promoting healthy circulation

Application:

Add a few drops of Lemon to water and white vinegar in a glass bottle to use as a disinfecting cleaning spray for kitchen counters and bathroom sinks. Apply directly to the skin for healing purposes (avoid exposure to the sun after use). Add a drop to a glass of water and drink it to give a boost to the immune system (of course you should only ingest oils that you know are 100% pure).

4. Eucalyptus Essential Oil

Eucalyptus radiata

The bright and somewhat medicinal scent of eucalyptus is minty with a hint of pine and sweetness. Some people describe the scent as sharp and clean, with a hint of camphor.

Useful for:

• Reducing congestion and stuffy noses

• Fighting germs (especially respiratory infections)

• Stimulating the mind and body

• Reducing fever

• Eliminating headaches

• Cooling

• Relief of muscle pain

• Insect repellent

• Boost immune system

Application:

At the first sign of a cold or flu, place a few drops of Eucalyptus essential oil in a diffuser and breathe it in to ward off winter infections and fight sinus congestion. Or add to a pot of hot water, place a towel over your head and inhale the steam. Add a few drops to a carrier oil and massage into tired and sore muscles.

5. Frankincense Essential Oil

Bosellia carterii

Known from ancient times as a precious commodity, Frankincense essential oil is extracted from the resin of a hardy tree. This oil is more expensive than many, and works well when blended with other oils to make it effective for a variety of reasons. The scent is woody and clean with a warm and spicy tone.

Useful for:

• Stress reduction

• Boosting immune system

• Killing germs and bacteria

• Healing skin and preventing signs of aging

• Improving mental clarity and memory

• Balancing hormones

• Aiding with digestion

• Promoting healthy sleep patterns

• Reducing swelling, inflammation, and pain

Application:

Diffuse into the air in winter months to kill germs and

boost your immune system. Apply directly to the skin on

the face before going to bed to keep the skin healthy, prevent wrinkles and fade dark spots. Or apply to warts, moles, and other skin problems. Take a deep sniff of this oil after eating a heavy meal to aid with digestion, or prior to going to sleep to help calm and relax.

6. Tea Tree Essential Oil

Melaleuca alternifolia

Another essential oil with a strong odor, tea tree oil is also commonly called 'Melaleuca'. This scent is very medicinal and acrid with a camphorous odor.

Useful for:

• Healing acne

• Treating athlete's foot and other fungal infections

• Reducing dandruff

• Treating bad breath and killing mouth germs.

• Insect repellent

• Congestion and cough due to cold

Application:

Apply directly to cuts, scrapes, and acne in order to kill germs and promote healthy healing. Add a drop to a glass of water and gargle to kill germs in the mouth. Dilute with a carrier oil and apply topically to skin affected by athlete's foot, nail fungus, or other infections.

7. Chamomile Essential Oil

Chamaemelum nobile

This oil has a sweet, flowery scent that some people compare to apple blossoms. It's an earthy, straw-like smell that many people find to be mild and enjoyable.

Useful for:

• Promoting relaxation and inducing sleep

• Lifting mood and relieving depression

• Fights bacteria (sores, acne, mouth)

• Soothes digestive problems

• Promote youthful looking skin and hair

Application:

Add a few drops to a cool mist humidifier and place in the bedroom to help calm and relax. Or add a few drops to a water bottle to create a pillow spray or room spray. Add a drop to your favorite herbal tea or apply directly to the abdomen to soothe digestive problems. Do not use if pregnant or breastfeeding.

8. Rosemary Essential Oil

Rosmarinus officinalis

This essential oil has a strongly herbal scent that has a mellow undertone reminiscent of camphor. If you don't like the scent, blend it with Peppermint or a citrus oil to cut the smell.

Useful for:

• Boosting memory and mental clarity

• Reducing congestion and sinus problems

• Soothing headaches

• Alleviating muscle pain and cramps

• Fighting against depression and anxiety

• Healing skin problems

• Aiding with healthy digestion

Application:

Add a few drops to a carrier oil and apply to the bottoms of the feet or abdomen to aid with digestion. Or apply to sore, achy muscles to help with pain. Place in a diffuser to bring a sense of peace and clarity to the room, reducing tension and fatigue. Do not use if pregnant or breastfeeding.

9. Patchouli Essential Oil

Pogostemon cablin

This is one of those scents that many people have to get used to as it is very earthy and pungent. Notorious for being used by hippies in the '60s and '70s, the scent is not always appreciated by everyone and can be blended with other oils to make it less obvious.

Useful for:

• Relieving anxiety

• Skin care and healing

• Reducing bloating

• Relaxation during massage

• Fighting depression

• Reducing fatigue

• Balancing hormones

Application:

Add a couple of drops to a carrier oil and apply directly to the face to keep your skin looking fresh and healthy. For grounding emotions, place a drop in the hand, cup the hand over the nose and mouth and breathe in naturally for a few minutes to receive the emotional and hormonal benefits.

10. Sweet Orange Essential Oil

Citrus sinensis

Popular and affordably priced, open a bottle of orange essential oil and the room will smell like you just peeled a fresh orange!

Useful for:

• Uplifting mood and easing anxiety

• Boosting immune system

• Preventing infection

• Aids in cognitive function

• Disinfecting households

• Reducing inflammation

• Decreasing hypertension

Application:

Add a few drops of orange essential oil to a spray bottle filled with water to use as a room freshening spray, counter disinfectant, or bathroom cleaner. Place a few drops of orange oil into a cool mist humidifier and diffuse into the room to boost moods, improve blood flow, and reduce stress.

11. Marjoram Essential Oil

Origanum marjorana

This oil made from the flowering marjoram plant has a slight 'green' scent that is similar to herbs such as thyme and cardamom, with a hint of peppery and camphor smells.

Useful for:

• Fighting fatigue

• Promoting healthy circulation

• Reducing constipation and cramps

• Calming hyperactive children

• Uplifting the mood

• Reducing tension and related headaches

• Relieving insomnia

• Reducing asthma symptoms

• Helping with healthy digestion

Application:

Add to a carrier oil and apply to the back of the neck to reduce feelings of stress and tension. Or apply, diluted, to the bottoms of the feet to promote heart health and have a positive effect on the nervous system. Diffuse into the room to soothe fussy children or calm anxious students. Not recommended if pregnant or breastfeeding.

12. Grapefruit Essential Oil

Citrus paradise or Citrus racemosa

Another oil from the popular citrus family, Grapefruit has an attractive scent that is energizing and affordably priced. Blend with spicy oils such as cinnamon for a balanced, warming atmosphere.

Useful for:

• Fighting jet lag

• Disinfecting bathrooms and kitchens

• Giving an energy boost

• Aiding with appetite suppression and weight loss

• Stimulating the immune system

• Reducing inflammation

Application:

Diffuse into the room to help balance emotions, boost energy, and suppress sugar cravings when trying to lose weight. Dilute in a carrier oil and apply topically for fighting throat and respiratory infections. Add to a spray bottle filled with water and white vinegar for a germ-fighting counter spray or bathroom cleanser.

13. Cinnamon Essential Oil

Cinnamomum zeylanicum

With a scent reminiscent of autumn, pumpkin pie spice, and warmth, cinnamon essential oil brings a cozy, comfortable atmosphere. The scent is especially enjoyable when blended with other spices (such as nutmeg and clove) or citrus oils like lemon and orange.

Useful for:

• Killing germs

• Treating headaches

• Calming negative thoughts

• Improving blood circulation

• Boosting brain function and clarity

• Helping with milk production in new mothers

• Maintaining a healthy immune system

• Relieving sore muscles and joints

Application:

Diffuse in the air to promote healthy blood flow to the brain and reduce headaches, as well as encouraging self-confidence and balancing emotions. Add a few drops to a carrier oil and apply directly to sore joints, or apply to the bottoms of the feet for pain relief throughout the body.

14. Clove Essential Oil

The scent of clove is strong and spicy, with a deep earthy tone that can be overpowering to some people. It is often blended with citrus or floral oils to tone down the scent.

Useful for:

• Reducing inflammation and swelling

• Relieving sore tooth or mouth pain

• Treating acne, cuts, or scrapes

• Reducing stress

• Treating headaches and sinus congestion

• Preventing or fighting infections

Application:

Add a drop to a glass of water and gargle for oral hygiene. Dilute with a carrier oil and apply topically to acne, boils, sores, rashes, or other skin problems. Apply, diluted, to the bottoms of the feet to promote good circulation, aid in digestion, eliminate toxins, and reduce inflammation or nausea.

15. Clary Sage Essential Oil

Salvia sclarea

This plant is not quite a well-known as some of the others, but its powerful benefits make it super popular as an essential oil. It does not smell like the commonly known cooking spice, called sage. The scent of this oil is earthy, herbal, balmy, and woody. Some people do not prefer the aroma and find it more tolerable when blended with lavender or other floral essential oils.

Useful for:

- Hormonal balance

- Fighting depression and reducing stress

- Relieving spasms and convulsions

- Preventing bacterial infections

- Promoting removal of free radicals and oxidants

- Reducing gas

- Caring for skin

- Regulating menstruation

- Lowering blood pressure

Application:

If you're a woman dilute with a carrier oil and apply directly to the abdomen and bottoms of the feet to help promote and stimulate regular menstruation in younger women and hormone balance in menopausal women. This same application on the feet can be used to calm nerves, lower blood pressure, and relieve depression. Apply, diluted, directly to the abdomen to reduce stomach disorders and relieve trapped gas. Use, diluted, as an anti-stress massage oil.

LEMONGRASS ESSENTIAL OIL USES

Lemongrass is one of my favorite essential oils. I like it best to get rid of nasty smells around the house. It is also a natural pesticide which drives away bugs and pests in the garden, allowing cultivation of other vegetables very convenient.

But that's not where this the power of this oil ends.

Have a look at these 13 ways you can use your bottle of Lemongrass oil.

COSMETIC

1. Lemongrass oil can be used as toner. Add one to two drops of essential oil to your regular cleanser or mix it with a hydrosol such as tea tree or lavender hydrosol, to dilute and make an effective skin toner. Apply to the skin using cotton rounds. Lemongrass is considered to be a milder extract, but don't use it undiluted. It can be too strong for sensitive skin.

2. It can also strengthen hair, promote hair growth, and relieve itching in the scalp. Mix few drops into your shampoo or conditioner. Its citrus essence promotes a

fresh feeling in the scalp. For best effects, use a natural, scent-free shampoo.

3. It can also be a good skin moisturizer. Mix a few drops of the essential oil with lotion or body gel.

MEDICINAL

4. Lemongrass oil is used to ease joint and muscle pain. It has pain-relieving properties that get rid of swelling, pain and other discomfort. Apply a diluted amount of Lemongrass onto the affected area and massage the muscles and joints. It soothes the muscles, and its relaxing scent promotes ease and relief. It is also a perfect way to cool down and relax muscles after a strenuous workout.

5. Because of its antiseptic property, lemongrass oil is beneficial in getting rid of bacteria and fungi. It can also

relieve swell and itch because of is astringent properties. Apply the essential oil topically to insect bites or dilute a few drops in carrier oil before applying to rashes or other skin irritations.

6. Lemongrass is also a natural pesticide in the garden. To protect your plants and greens. It's safe to use daily.

7. The antibacterial property of the lemongrass oil allows it to be used in soaps and sanitizers. Soap and sanitizers sold commercially sometimes have lemongrass essences.

8. Aromatic air fresheners use lemongrass oil to relieve insomnia and anxiety which promotes better sleep. Use 4-5 drops of lemongrass essential oil in your diffuser. Diffusing it in your car or room creates an enjoyable ambiance of pure freshness and relaxation.

9. Lemongrass oil can be used as an insect repellent. Its strong and distinct smell can repel insects like mosquitoes and bugs so it is a very good travel essential. Mix it in with your perfume, lotion or you can also opt to diffuse it with an aromatherapy bracelet. If you prefer to camp, you can dilute a few drops of oil in water and spray your tent to ward off unwanted insects.

10. When having stomach troubles, massage this essential oil onto the belly to relieve bloating. One to two drops of this essential oil can help you soothe stomach pain caused by excess gas, ulcer and upset stomach. Use 1 teaspoon of carrier oil, and 1-2 drops of Lemongrass.

THERAPEUTIC

11. Lemongrass oil has that distinct fresh and citrus-like aroma that opens up nasal airways and creates a relaxed

feeling. Use Lemongrass to make deodorizers and sanitizers. It has been widely used in spas as it creates a fresh and calming ambiance. It also deodorizes and gets rid of unpleasant smells. A few drops in the diffuser will go a long way.

12. The aromatic smell of lemongrass oil can relieve stress and anxiety. It is essential in aromatherapy because of its positive effect on the body. It promotes soothing and calming feeling. A few drops in the diffuser is all that's needed.

13. Lemongrass oil can also relieve nausea. Drop one to two drops into a cotton ball or handkerchief. Take a deep breath in. Allow the scent to penetrate the nasal passage. Or, make a roll-on and massage your temples and forehead.

The Importance of Using Botanical Names with Essential Oils

A plant's common name is the name that we casually use to refer to a botanical. Examples of common names include Eucalyptus, Orange, Chamomile and Bay.

As is the case with each of these examples, however, different plants can sometimes share the same common name. For example, there are several types of Chamomile. This can be highly problematic because plants sharing the same common name don't necessarily share the same therapeutic properties, benefits or contraindications.

To eliminate this confusion and the unfortunate problems that can arise from it, "botanical nomenclature" is used to systematically name plants in Latin so that no two plants share the same Latin name that is assigned to the plant.

Within the scope of essential oils and holistic aromatherapy, the unique names assigned to plants are typically known as "botanical names" or "Latin names." The first word is known as the Genus, and it should be capitalized. The second word is the species and should appear in all lowercase letters. The entire botanical name should be italicized.

Botanical Name Examples

Lemon: Citrus limon

Peppermint: Mentha piperita

Pink Pepper: Schinus molle

Tea Tree: Melaleuca alternifolia

The Use of Botanical Names When Referring to and Shopping for Essential Oils

When you shop for essential oils or refer to resources, it's important to pay attention to the botanical name of the essential oil that you are interested in. For example, if you're reading a profile pertaining to Sweet Orange Essential Oil you will notice that the corresponding botanical name for Sweet Orange Essential Oil is Citrus sinensis. If you decide you want to research Sweet Orange Essential Oil further and possibly purchase it, you will want to be sure to doublecheck the botanical name listed for any Orange Oil that you are considering purchasing, even if it is listed as Sweet Orange Essential Oil. Sweet Orange Essential Oil is not phototoxic, but Bitter Orange Essential Oil is phototoxic.

Not only is it important to ensure that you are working with the correct essential oil for safety and therapeutic reasons, but it's also important from a conservation perspective. Some essential oil oil bearing plants and trees like Atlas Cedarwood (Cedrus atlantica) are endangered yet Virginian Cedardwood (Juniperus virginiana) is not. Therefore, Juniperus virginiana is the better choice from a mindful, sustainability perspective.

When you shop, doublecheck the botanical names to help ensure that you don't accidentally purchase the wrong essential oil for your needs. If a supplier does not provide the botanical name of an essential oil, be leery. Most all reputable sellers realize the importance and necessity of including the botanical name on their bottle labels and marketing materials. For the sake of brevity it's standard practice and acceptable for essential oil educators and authors to only use the common name if they link the common name to a page that includes the botanical name or if they provide the botanical name somewhere else within easy access to the reader/student.

As I mentioned above, botanical nomenclature is a naming system used so that no two plants share the same botanical name. However, botanical nomenclature can change over time, and there are some plants that are known by more than one botanical name. For example, Lavendula officinalis used to be the preferred botanical name for Lavender Essential Oil. Now the preferred botanical name is Lavandula angustifolia, but both botanical names for Lavender are still in use.

STORING ESSENTIAL OILS

Why Does Essential Oil Storage Matter?

Proper essential oil storage can drastically protect and prolong the shelf life of your oils. The type of glass your oils are stored in, the temperature they are stored at and the sun beaming down on your essential oil bottles can all impact their quality.

This focuse primarily upon storing essential oils to maximumize their shelf life, but it is also important that you remember that essential oils should be stored so that they cannot be accessed by children or those who may not understand how to use them safely. Essential oils are flammable, so careful storage away from heat and fire sources is also important.

How to Store Essential Oils to Maximize Their Shelf Life

For individual use, essential oils, absolutes and CO2s are most often sold in 5ml, 10ml and 15ml (1/2 ounce) sizes. For more expensive oils, it is common to find them available in sizes starting at 2ml and 1 dram sizes.

Although essential oils do not become rancid, they do oxidize, deteriorate and lose their beneficial therapeutic properties over time. Oils such as the citrus oils will oxidize and begin to lose their aroma and therapeutic properties in as little as six months. Not all essential oils diminish in aromatic quality as time passes. The aroma of essential oils such as patchouli and sandalwood mature with age, however, all essential oils oxidize and are subject to losing their therapeutic value in time. All essential oils benefit from proper storage and handling.

To avoid deterioration and protect the aromatic and therapeutic properties of your essential oils, store them in amber or cobalt blue bottles. Dark glass such as amber or cobalt helps to keep out deteriorating sunlight. It is best not to store essential oils in clear glass bottles. Clear glass bottles are not harmful to essential oils, but clear glass does not protect the oils from damaging sunlight. In comparison, you may have noticed that most bottled beer typically is packaged in amber (brown) glass bottles to help protect the contents from exposure to light. Except for certain situations that most often pertain for bulk oil purchases, avoid purchasing or storing pure essential oils in plastic bottles as the essential oil will eat at the plastic, and the essential oil will become ruined over a short period of time. Some vendors sell oils in lined aluminum bottles. It has been said that aluminum bottles are acceptable if the interior of the bottles are lined.

Essential oils should also be stored in a cool, dark place.

Avoid purchasing essential oils that are stored in bottles that have a rubber dropper incorporated into its screw-top cap. Droppers with rubber bulbs should not be kept with the essential oil bottle as the highly concentrated oil can turn the rubber bulb into gum and ruin the essential oil.

Instead of a rubber dropper top, many essential oils that are sold to consumers in sizes of 1 ounce (30 ml) and smaller are packaged in bottles that contain an orifice reducer. An orifice reducer is a small, clear insert inside the bottle opening that acts as a built-in dropper. They are also known as euro droppers. Unlike the material that rubber dropper bulbs are made of, orifice reducers are made of a material that can withstand exposure to essential oils. The name orifice reducer may seem a little strange at first, but it's a handy little dispensing device. You simply tip the bottle and you can dispense the oil drop by drop.

Not all essential oil suppliers provide orifice reducers. This is not necessarily a reflection on the integrity of the company or the quality of their oils. Wholesalers in particular often do not package with orifice reducers as their primary clientele are artisans and larger natural/holistic formulators that don't dispense essential oils by the drop. If this is important to you, it's best to ask vendors what type of packaging they use when bottling their oils.

Store Your Essential Oils in a Cool Location or the Refrigerator

Store essential oils in a refrigerated environment, whenever possible. If that is not possible, store them in as cool a location as possible.

HOW TO USE ESSENTIAL OILS FOR

HAIR & SKIN CARE

• Body Spray

In a spray bottle, combine 5 to 10 drops of an essential oil and 4 ounces of water and shake. If you choose citrus oil, be careful when applying it near your face. Some citrus oils may be phototoxic or photosensitizers, making your skin more susceptible to sunburn.

• Shampoo

Support the health of your scalp by adding a few drops of lavender, cedarwood or basil to your shampoo. Try adding rosemary oil to your shampoo to boost volume and increase circulation in the scalp.

• Skin cream

Add two drops of rosemary oil to your skin cream for antioxidant support and protection against oxidative stress.

• Make your own body oil

Add up to 5 drops of an essential oil to a teaspoon of carrier oil, such as sweet almond, olive, apricot kernel, borage seed, jojoba, sesame, sunflower or wheat germ oil.

• Add to your hot tub or bathwater

Add up to 6 drops of essential oils to ¼ cup of your favorite carrier oil (we like jojoba oil) before adding 8 to 10 drops of the blended oils to a bath. Avoid culinary oils including cinnamon, lemongrass and peppermint as they can cause skin irritations.

Which Essential Oil Can Support the Health of Your Hair?

Not only is lavender a perennial favorite among aromatherapists, but research also shows that it can support hair health when used regularly to massage the scalp. Here's a quick at-home, step-by-step lavender massage guide for your hair and scalp:

1. Warm about half a cup of olive oil (not too hot).

2. Blend in about 10 drops (or to your preference) of lavender oil.

3. Apply this blend to your hair and gently massage your scalp.

4. Wrap a warm towel around your head, sit back and relax for about 20 minutes.

5. Follow it up with a natural shampoo and conditioner.

Best for Sleep and Self Care

Use Lavender oil in baths, sprays, lotions, oils and more as a part of your bedtime ritual since lavender may promote a calm and relaxed feeling. Make a quick lavender-scented pillow insert by adding 3 drops of lavender oil to a wash cloth or linen square and placing it inside your pillow case. Make your own calming body oil by adding 3 to 5 drops of lavender oil to 2 tablespoons of a carrier oil like sweet almond or jojoba oil to support skin health and relaxation, especially during the dry winter months.

How to Use Essential Oils for Home & Hearth

• Deter pests

Place one drop of lavender oil on a cotton ball or piece of cloth to help temporarily get rid of moths and mosquitoes.

• Humidifiers

To help keep your humidifier smelling fresh, add up to 9 drops of tea tree oil.

• Fire logs

Thirty minutes before burning a fire log, place one drop of cypress, pine, sandalwood or cedarwood oil on it. Do not use several perfumed logs at a time; a little goes a long way.

• Stuffed animals

Soothe your kids with the calming scent of lavender or chamomile on their stuffed animals. Place a stuffed animal in a plastic bag, add a few drops of essential oil and close the plastic bag overnight. The following day the stuffed animal will have the dispersed scent and can be used for up to two weeks before reapplying more oil.

Best for Freshening Your Home

Lemon oil or Eucalyptus oil are best to help freshen your home and provide an invigorating, refreshing, and cleansing scent. Select one oil or use both: add 2 drops to a dryer ball to freshen your laundry or 4 drops to an ultrasonic diffuser to help freshen your home with an energizing scent.

Tip: For maximum effectiveness, use essential oils within one year of opening the bottle.

Essential Oils Carpet Refresher Recipe

This is a brilliant way to freshen up your house by using essential oils. Add your favorite scent to your rooms while you freshen your carpets with this simple mixture that costs pennies to make.

In a large bowl, combine 1 cup of baking soda or cornstarch with 7-10 drops of essential oil. Break up any clumps with a fork and stir well. Pour mixture into a cheese shaker or can with holes punched into the lid. Sprinkle liberally over the carpet. Wait 30 minutes, then vacuum.

Essential Oils for a Natural Bug Spray

Making your own natural bug spray at home is easy. A natural bug spray may provide temporary relief from bugs, but keep in mind they require more frequent application and higher concentrations than some commercial repellants. Sunscreens, sweat, water and evaporation from wind or high temperatures can lower effectiveness.

Essential Oil Safety

Essential oils are highly concentrated, and they can be harmful if not used carefully. Implementing aromatherapy into your lifestyle shouldn't cause paranoia or undue worry, but it is important to learn about and heed essential oil safety. By treating essential oils with respect and learning about essential oil safety, you will be well on your way to safely enjoying the many benefits that essential oils can offer.

These safety guidelines are intended as a helpful introduction, but they should not be considered a complete safety reference for the proper use of essential oils.

• It is safest to consult with a qualified medical or aromatherapy practitioner before implementing essential oils into your lifestyle.

• Essential oils should never be used undiluted on the skin. Lavender and tea tree are listed by a large number of aromatherapy sources as being oils that can be used undiluted. Undiluted use of lavender and tea tree, however, should be discouraged as severe sensitivity still could occur in some individuals. Again, the safest rule of thumb is to never use any essential oil undiluted and to be sure to dilute all essential oils adequately.

• Some oils can cause irritation, sensitization or allergic reactions in some individuals. When using a new oil topically for the first time, do a skin patch test on a small area of skin (it's easy).

• Some essential oils are phototoxic and can cause irritation, inflammation, blistering, redness and/or burning when exposed to UVA rays.

• Discontinue using an essential oil or essential oil blend immediately if you encounter any irritation, redness or reaction.

• Using essential oils in the bath requires special care. Never add essential oils directly to bathwater.

• Some essential oils should be avoided during pregnancy or by those with asthma, epilepsy, or with other health conditions.

• Be sure to research/review the safety precautions associated with each essential oil that you use.

• Less IS More. When using essential oils, use the smallest amount of essential oil that will get the job done. If 1-2 drops are called for, for example, don't use more than that. Essential oils are very concentrated. (As a sidenote, some companies or their representatives may suggest that you use as much as you want – it's in their best interest that you go through your oils faster so you then need to reorder more frequently. Generally speaking, it takes a lot of plant material (i.e. flower petals, leaves, needles, bark, wood, root, etc.) to obtain the botanical's essential oil by steam distillation. It's wasteful to use more essential oil than is needed for your particular application.)

• Not all essential oils are suitable for use in aromatherapy. Wormwood, pennyroyal, onion, camphor, horseradish, wintergreen, rue, bitter almond and sassafras are examples of some of the essential oils that should only be used by qualified aromatherapy practitioners, if ever at all.

• Essential oils oxidize over time and can become more sensitizing/irritating. Avoid using old or improperly stored essential oils for therapeutic applications.

• Avoid using essential oils near the genitals, mouth, nose, eyes and ears.

• Essential oils do not stay mixed with water and should never be added to bathwater without first being diluted/solubilized. Essential oils that are at higher risk of causing irritation and sensitization should be avoided in the bath, even if you solubilize them.

• Use extreme caution when using oils with children or the elderly. Be sure to first read the recommended dilution ratios for children.

• Never let children use essential oils without the presence of an adult knowledgeable about their use. Most essential oils smell wonderful and many essential oils such as citrus oils can smell like they are "yummy" and safe to drink. ALWAYS keep your essential oils away from children. Treat the oils like medicines that are poison in unknowing hands.

• The same essential oils and blends that we use on ourselves are not always safe to use on our dogs, cats, birds, horses or other pets.

• Diffuse essential oils sensibly. They should not be continuously diffused. Be sure you are diffusing in a well ventilated space.

• Essential oils should not be taken internally without guidance by a qualified practitioner or until you have gained adequate knowledge and understanding of the risks and safe internal applications and dosages. Even though essential oils are cold pressed or steam distilled from a range of citrus and common spices like Lemons, Oranges, Grapefruits, Allspice, Basil, Black Pepper, Cinnamon, Clove, Fennel, Ginger, Rosemary and a number of other botanicals that are routinely ingested without the need for precautionary usage info, essential oils are highly concentrated and should not be ingested without thorough understanding of appropriate usage and risks for each oil.

• Essential oils are flammable. Keep them out of the way of fire hazards.